i

The

21st Century

FAT SWITCH

Burn fat easily and improve body shape! The easy programme for men and women to lose weight and improve health, without cutting calories or going hungry!

Michael Littlewood Dip GM, Dip SDT Nutritionist

Disclaimer

All the material contained in this book is provided for educational and informational purposes only. No responsibility can be taken for any results or outcomes resulting from the use of this material.

While every attempt has been made to provide information that is both accurate and effective, the author does not assume any responsibility for the accuracy or use/misuse of this information.

Medical Disclaimer

This information is not a substitute for proper medical advice, you should consult your doctor before making any dietary changes or taking up any exercise.

About the Author

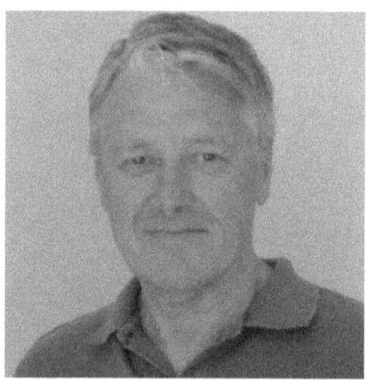

Michael Littlewood Dip GM, Dip SDT

Author, Nutritionist and Self Development Trainer

Michael Littlewood is a qualified Nutritionist and Personal Development Trainer.

He has worked for the UK NHS as a Health Trainer and has managed the Adult Weight Management on Referral Program, helping hundreds of people to successfully lose weight, many with related health problems.

To support The 21st Century Fat Switch programme he has a range of health, weight loss, fitness and wellbeing products available through his website and discount online store at **alphapeople.co.uk** and **taowarrior.co.uk**

Preface

Why are we all finding it so difficult to lose FAT when you can get great results in only 7 days?

This book explains The 21st Century FAT SWITCH, you can now just turn it off and still eat great healthy food with no calorie counting!

I use the word FAT deliberately because it is the FAT we want to lose not the muscle which gives our body shape and structure.

Learn how to get your body to Burn FAT and increase Energy by lowering Insulin levels.

Prevent more FAT being deposited and retain healthy muscle.

The key to The 21st Century FAT SWITCH is **lower Insulin!** How's it work?

Put simply, Insulin causes the body to deposit excess carbohydrate as FAT, particularly around the waist and hips and it prevents existing body fat from being used for energy.

By lowering Insulin levels you are throwing the **FAT SWITCH** not only do you prevent more fat being gained but you switch on your bodies fat burning mechanism.

So you automatically BURN FAT - NOT DEPOSIT FAT.

Stay with me and I will show you how!

Table   of   Contents

Chapter 1: Introduction

This book shows you how to lose fat in just seven days, without starving yourself and how to adapt eating habits to keep that going until you are at your desired weight! It includes not only a complete easy program to help you lose weight but clear, well informed advice to assist in health improvement, it just requires a bit of effort for great results.

It works because the changes are in the key most effective area of weight loss and health improvement, This is **Insulin Reduction.** The changes are simple, quick to follow and they will fit into any lifestyle.

Very soon these changes become normal to you, they become your habit and you will not see yourself as being on a diet at all.

This is for people who don't want to fast, starve themselves, feel constantly hungry, spend all day exercising, counting calories or obsessing about food, it's for people who love life and want to get on with it!

This book contains full supporting information for meat eaters and vegetarians, alternatives are also listed for those on special diets. The advice in this book has been developed from my experience as a

National Health Service (NHS) Health Trainer and from running the NHS Adult Weight Management Program in my County. Additionally I have incorporated the latest effective weight loss and nutritional science to give you control over what will work for you.

The people already successfully following our program are testimony to how enjoyable and do-able it is. We have made it clear and easy to follow, with lots of support, your biggest challenge will probably be readiness to change and you are here, reading this, wanting to do something, wanting change, so clearly you are ready!

When weight loss occurs it is not only undesirable fat that is lost but a significant proportion of muscle mass and bone density. The Fat Switch addresses this and can not only enable you to lose dangerous and unwanted fat whilst retaining muscle mass and bone density but can enable you to actually build muscle, strengthen bones and improve nutrition. In fact we will set out to reverse damage previously caused by slightly increasing your protein and calcium intake! This can be made very straightforward by taking a good quality protein shake as part of your routine. As you journey through the program we will clearly explain how this is done and why this level of health is essential for avoiding disease and maintaining vitality and a high quality life.

This does not need to be expensive, we will advise you on nutrition and how to identify cheap healthy foods you can introduce into your lifestyle. At the same time we will dispel advertising myths and advise you on how to identify foods that have little or no nutritional value or that may even be causing your problems!

Chapter 2: Why The 21st Century Fat Switch Works

The Fat Switch is based on established medical science with the addition of our cutting edge advanced nutritional knowledge and for many of you may only involve a few simple yet key changes to your diet and lifestyle.

Our diet in the western world has become mostly carbohydrate based, that is, we are very dependent on bread, cereals, rice, pasta, potatoes and highly processed food for our energy.

When we eat processed carbohydrates or sugary food we cause the body to produce **Insulin** to lower the blood sugar, the greater the volume or the more sweet the carbs, the more insulin is released.

This is bad for TWO very important reasons:

1. Any carbs that the insulin cannot deal with will be "parked as FAT", deposited as FAT especially around the waist and hips.

2. As long as insulin is present your body is prevented from using FAT deposits to provide energy, so you can NEVER burn FAT if insulin levels are high!

Understand this and you understand why we all get progressively fatter, whatever we try to do!

HIGH CARBS = HIGH INSULIN = FAT BUILDUP AND NO BURN

The really good news is that if we lower our carb intake we lower our insulin levels, not only do we stop laying down so much fat but we activate our body to BURN BODY FAT as its first option for energy production!

How do we set out to do this? We **THROW THE FAT SWITCH!**

Chapter 3: Let's throw that Fat Switch!

It is important to note this is not a starvation diet! With starvation diets you lose weight but not FAT! We are going to **retain or even increase strength, energy, muscle mass and bone density.**

I suggest that at the beginning of this journey you consider taking a photo of yourself, many people find this very motivational and a reminder of just how far they have come!

We split the changes into two phases:

FAT Loss and **Weight Maintenance**, you choose how long you stay on the Fat loss phase but I suggest an initial 7 days to establish how well its working for you.

In the FAT Loss phase we replace poor quality refined carbs with healthier food from other food groups to make sure you are not hungry. We are going to virtually cut out all refined carbohydrates, a table is provided listing these but broadly they are sugar, sweets, cakes, biscuits, white flour, white rice and pasta. We will replace these with better carbohydrates, also listed but limit our intake to around **50 grams per day**. This is very important to throw the fat switch!

In the Weight Maintenance phase you increase your better

carbohydrate intake to around **100 grams per day** but you have learnt to recognise and avoid poor quality high GI carbs. You can with practice, find your own level, one that works naturally for you and gives easy weight loss or weight maintenance. In time this will just become the way you eat and will not seem at all like a diet at all.

I have given you good meal ideas that fit into both phases for breakfast, lunch and dinner plus healthy snack suggestions. Choosing from either the tables or the meal menus will work for you and later in the book is more in depth information on nutrition and the other food groups. You have probably noticed that I have not mention calories yet, that is because **we are not counting calories**. You will get all the calories you need each day by switching to other nutritious, healthy and tasty foods like protein, meat and fish, good fats, vegetables, salads, seeds and nuts.

I am not in favour of strict rules for diets, we want to keep this do-able, so the **50 grams per day limit** is a recommendation, use the Daily Carbohydrate Record Table to help you keep track. This will tell you what you have left for your evening meal. Print a few of these off for yourself and keep them with you, to stay in control.

You should monitor your own energy levels and your own weight loss and body change. As long as you understand the Fat Switch principle and do your best, it should work for you. However, if whatever you have been doing has created your current position you will have to make changes! **Now go for it and learn as you go!**

Vital Reminder 1

Any carbs that the insulin cannot deal with will be "parked as FAT",

Vital Reminder 2

As long as insulin is present your body is prevented from using FAT deposits

Your Daily Carbohydrate Record Table

Record all the grams of carbs you eat at each meal or snack and add them up to stay within 50 grams daily for the weight loss phase

Carbohydrate Choices Description. Your target in Fat Loss phase is 50 grams, 100 grams in Weight Maintenance phase	Portion size if known	Grams of Carbs

Chapter 4: Start with a Low Carbohydrate Breakfast

Breakfast is an important meal and should not be skipped. Missing breakfast is likely to lead to grabbing the wrong kind of snack later in the morning. In fact missing meals at all causes the body to release a hormone called **ghrelin** which indirectly causes you to really want high calorie, high fat foods. This would increase insulin levels and prevent our Fat Switch from working for us, so the bottom line is:

EAT THREE REGULAR MEALS A DAY!

Now for another shock!

All cereals should be thrown out immediately! They mostly are fast release (High GI) and very high in carbs, often with added sugar, raising insulin levels very quickly, they will also leave you hungry again within a couple of hours. Just one bowl of average cereals with milk and a spoon of sugar add up to around 55 grams of carbohydrates, blowing your new diet immediately!

Key Point

Cereals are mostly very refined
Carbs with added sugar, so are
fast release. Avoid them!

Are you shocked yet?   Well hear this!

Fruit juices and smoothies are out during the weight loss phase!

I hear you say "but these are healthy", well yes they are a source of antioxidants, vitamins and fibre, but many fruits are naturally high in sugars, which are carbohydrates and turning them into juice can change them from slow release to medium release. This again causes insulin levels to rise quickly so you will have to limit fruit and avoid fruit juices during this weight loss phase. Happily, Figs at just 5 grams of carbs and Kiwi Fruit at 6 grams with fresh yogurt, can contribute to a great breakfast.

Key Point

Fruit juices and smoothies are high in sugar and are fast release. Avoid them!

See the table for more, low carb fruit choices.

These are a few ideas for a good breakfast with the number of grams shown so that you can keep track, if you don't see anything you like simply replace with items from the low carbohydrate table that follows. Experiment and have fun. Be unconventional about breakfast and stick to the guidance, avoiding highly processed, fast release foods

Table: Good Breakfast Ideas

Good breakfast ideas	Usual Portion Size	Grams of Carbs
Poached egg on wholemeal toast with butter	88 grams	16 grams
Porridge made with milk and water	160 grams	14 grams
Two egg omelette	120 grams	0 grams
Fresh Fig or Kiwi Fruit, fresh double cream	100 grams	7 grams
Gouda cheese, butter, on melba toast (2)	80 grams	8 grams
Field mushroom, cream cheese, omelette	150 grams	1 gram
Smoked salmon and cream cheese	130 grams	1 gram
Smoked salmon and scrambled eggs (2)	200 grams	1 gram
Fried egg and bacon	160 grams	0 grams
Poached eggs (2) and spinach in garlic	190 grams	1 gram
Sausage, egg, bacon, tomato	200 grams	3 grams
Cheese omelette	180 grams	1 gram
Haloumi, tomatoes, bacon, garlic mushrooms	160 grams	0 grams
Kipper grilled with poached egg	200 grams	0 grams

Table: Low Carbohydrate Breakfast Alternatives

Low Carbohydrate Breakfast Alternatives mix and match for a great breakfast Description	Usual Portion Size	Grams of Carbs
Grilled gammon rashers	100 grams	0 grams
Tinned ham sliced	100 grams	0 grams
Bacon rashers	100 grams	0 grams
Corned beef	100 grams	2 grams
Sausages, pork or beef, grilled	60 grams	6 grams
Field mushroom	80 grams	0 grams
Yogurt, natural, Greek style	150 grams	7 grams
Cottage cheese	60 grams	1 gram
Cream cheese	50 grams	1 gram
Paneer	60 grams	1 gram
Mozzarella cheese	80 grams	1 gram
Red Leicester cheese	60 grams	1 gram
Fried egg , olive oil	60 grams	0 grams
Smoked Salmon	80 grams	0 grams

Use the 7 week record card to record your weekly progress or make a copy and keep it going, record your energy level and how you feel about yourself on a scale of 1 to 10 and watch for improvement particularly around your waist!

Let's get started, fill in the first line of your card.

Your 7 week record card

Week Start Date	Weight Pounds or Kilos	Waist Size Inches or Cms	Measure of Health and Energy 1 to 10

Chapter 5: You will NOT starve!

Medical science widely accepts that to lose weight at 1 to 2 pounds a week you must reduce your calorie intake by around 600 calories per day. However we now know this is ignoring the effects of The Fat Switch which we are going to get to work in your favour. By following The Fat Switch your calories will reduce automatically, so no need to think about calories at all, carbs are the key to your weight loss.

Reminder

As long as insulin is present your body is prevented from using FAT deposits to provide energy.

We also know that the quality of those calories is critical to your health and we will address this in more detail in later chapters. For now let's establish how many grams of carbohydrates that you should be aiming to take in, to get that weight loss started. You can be assured at this stage that the recommendations in the Good Breakfast Table and

Alternatives Table are healthy and balanced.

Diets that severely restrict what you can eat are not sustainable in the long term and drastically limiting calories as a lifestyle may be effectively starving you of essential nutrition. We will not starve you! Life is to be enjoyed and we are looking to create that new level of energy and vitality, in fact a new you! The latest research supports the fact that simply reducing calories does not work. In fact some diets leave your body so depleted in essential nutrition that serious and permanent damage can be caused.

I have allowed some flexibility around the 50 gram target because women and men have different metabolic rates (the rate at which your body burns calories). Your metabolic rate also slows down with age so you will find it necessary to allow for this and keep an eye on your own energy levels, we are all different and unique! Simply follow the guidelines and find what works for you and creates weight loss over the first seven day period, then adjust your carbs if necessary. It may seem that you are eating less but this is made up by the nutritious increase in protein, fats and vegetables that also provide a slower release of energy, keeping you feeling satisfied for longer.

So be assured that you will not starve and every factor is starting to work for you!

Next follows some poor Carbohydrate choices, which means they are high in Carbs or fast release (High GI). Your body could struggle to deal with these in a manageable way, raise insulin levels quickly and will lay down FAT!

Reminder

**Break the habit of grabbing
highly refined carbs it causes a
rush of insulin and deposits
FAT!**

Your Refined Carbs Table

Avoid these quick release carbohydrates!

Poor Carbohydrate Choices avoid these Description	Usual Portion Size	Grams of Carbs
white bread, baguette, rolls	40 grams	25 grams
White rice, brown rice, pasta	180 grams	55 grams
Jacket potato	200 grams	58 grams
Chips or any pizza	170 grams	50 grams
Pastries, pies and cakes	60 grams	38 grams
Fast food, burgers, hot dogs, wraps	200 grams	40 grams
Faggots in gravy	150 grams	19 grams
Quiche	140 grams	24 grams
Potato curry, chickpea curry	220 grams	30 grams
Sweet potato	140 grams	37 grams
Bean salad	190 grams	25 grams
Colas, carbonated drinks and fruit juices	160 grams	16 grams
Biscuits	26 grams	18 grams

Corn Flakes, mueslis and most cereals	45 grams	30 grams

Your Better Carbs Table

Limit yourself to 50 grams in weight loss phase!

Better Carbohydrate choices Description	Usual Portion Size	Grams of Carbs
Cod or haddock in batter	170 grams	20 grams
Roasted quarter chicken	150 grams	0 grams
Tomato juice	160 grams	5 grams
Coffee with cream	190 grams	1 gram
Chinese tea, green tea or herbal tea	190 grams	0 grams
Pork pie, pork and egg pie	60 grams	10 grams
Almonds, Brazil nuts, Walnuts	20 grams	1 gram
Melon seeds, sunflower seeds, pine nuts	15 grams	2 grams
Liver pate, mackerel pate	40 grams	2 grams
Peanut butter, smooth or crunchy	25 grams	2 grams
Boiled egg	50 grams	6 grams
Cream cheese	35 grams	1 gram
Stir fried vegetables	300 grams	6 grams

Prawns, shelled	120 grams	0 grams

Chapter 6: Lunch at last!

You have eaten a good breakfast and now it is lunch time at last and if you ate a breakfast from the list or improvised sensibly you will have got here without having to snack on sugary food mid-morning. That is because the food choices were low carb and low GI so the slow release of energy sustained you for two to three hours rather than eating a bowl of cereals and being hungry again in an hour.

If you didn't make it all the way I hope you managed to snack sensibly from the choices given on the Good Snack Table. Don't beat yourself up as you are changing well embedded habits and routines that may take a bit of time to become your new normal routine!

The best way to provide yourself with a good, nutritious lunch is to follow the boy scout motto and "BE PREPARED". If you can pack a lunch box at home you have control over your choices, think PROTEIN, SALAD or VEGETABLES chopped, FATS and a small amount of carbs. Here's the good news, your PROTEIN, that is, meat, fish, seafood cheese, tofu etc. can be up to TWICE what you would normally consider a serving because **protein will keep you satisfied for longer**.

So being prepared is the best way, but if you can't you will notice that most of the lunch options you have available to you are carbohydrate based. Examples are things like sandwiches and rolls, subway rolls, burgers, pizza, pasta, cereal bars and wraps. These will often be labelled as "Healthy Option" or "Low Fat", **don't be fooled!** Now we know what to look for, take a look at the **carbohydrates** on the label and get them as low as possible. You are looking for protein and fat which are nutritious and will keep you satisfied longer, things like humous, peanut butter, nuts, cream cheese, a tin of tuna or other fish and low carb rye cracker with as much salad as you like. If a sandwich really is the only option, go for wholegrain and take off the top slice of bread, you now have an open sandwich and you have just halved the fast release carbs!

The same with a Subway or similar sandwich bar, get loads of filling and leave most of the bread, people will think you are crazy but you don't have to eat it just because it has been put in front of you!

You can treat a wrap in the same way, eat the bit that holds the filling in and leave the fold at the bottom, it's the filling that has the nutrition, the rest has no nutritional value. If you need a boost have half a tub or more of protein like humous or cream cheese with your open sandwich and you will be satisfied. I usually carry two or three oat cakes for when I am out and just go for salad and protein, for me this is now normal and I certainly don't feel deprived in any way. Having a low carbohydrate protein shake with you is another good standby but watch out for those carbs, sugars and sweeteners.

If you are having a larger meal at lunchtime get into the habit of ordering carefully, think "Protein and salad or vegetable", so salmon or steak could be a great choice, just leave the chips or potatoes and do NOT go for a jacket potato as this is a fast release carbohydrate. Have a salad with your meat, fish or cheese, or peas and beans which are also a protein sources.

Familiarise yourself with the ideas in the table, think about the content of your meal, enjoy your lunch, don't skip it. Simply top up with nuts or seeds if you really are still hungry.

Reminder

Protein keeps you fuller, longer and helps maintain muscle and bone density!

Table: Good Lunch Ideas

Good Lunch Ideas Think protein, salad or green vegetables	Usual Portion Size	Grams of Carbs
Spanish omelette	150 grams	9 grams
Pork pie with salad	60 grams	11 grams
Two egg omelette with salad	120 grams	13 grams
Chicken, cashew and vegetable stir fry	340 grams	9 grams
Cream cheese and salad	60 grams	2 grams
Sirloin steak and salad	180 grams	0 grams
Smoked salmon, cream cheese, melba toast	100 grams	4 grams
Pork and egg pie with salad	60 grams	10 grams
Pate and salad	60 grams	3 grams
Greek style natural yoghurt	150 grams	7 grams
Corned beef and salad	100 grams	2 grams
Chicken drumsticks (2)	145 grams	14 grams
Seafood cocktail	100 grams	4 grams
Grilled kebab	100 grams	0 carbs

Chapter 7: Your Evening Meal

Now it's the end of the day you have done well with your breakfast, lunch and snacks, hopefully you have avoided refined carbohydrates and your good carb choices are within range. Check your record of the number of carbs you have consumed so far during the day to see how many carbs are left for you to keep under 50 grams.

The principles here are just the same, think low carbs, slow release carbs and lots of protein, salad or veg. This is your chance to really prepare something great for yourself or even if you are not a great cook keep it fresh, plain and wholesome. Stir frying is a tasty and good way to prepare food, using olive oil, garlic and Five Spice, it is one of my standby meals. With lots of veg, cashews and quorn or chicken you find you do not even need to add any carbs at all .

I promised I would make this easy, so you don't have to cook different meals to normal, simply reduce the carbohydrate part of your meals and increase the vegetables and protein. Eating at home gives you most control but if you are eating out the next chapter has a few ideas on staying within your diet goals without missing out.

Motivation Booster

Producing less Insulin gives you
more energy and keeps you
younger!

Table: Ideas for Evening Meals

Evening Meal Ideas Protein, salad and your allowed carbs!	Usual Portion Size	Grams of Carbs
Stir fried beef with green peppers in sauce	360 grams	11 grams
Mussels in shells	40 grams	1 gram
Two egg omelette	120 grams	13 grams
Prawns boiled and shelled	60 grams	1 gram
Grilled rainbow trout	155 grams	0 grams
Grilled salmon	80 grams	0 grams
Roast duck	185 grams	O grams
Chicken Korma	350 grams	8 grams
Lamb rogan josh	350 grams	6 grams
Green chicken curry	350 grams	5 grams
Chicken satay	170 grams	5 grams
Turkey grilled or roasted	90 grams	0 grams
Vegeburger or bean burger	60 grams	4 grams
Cauliflower cheese	200 grams	10 grams

Chapter 8: Eating out

You may think that eating out is going to be difficult but most restaurants these days are pleased to meet the special requirements of their customers. Almost every menu will include a number of dishes that will fall within our low carb guidelines. If this is not the case ask that the carbs be left out or alternatively just don't eat them.

You can see from the Evening Meal Ideas Table that it may be easier than you think, if you eat fish, turkey, duck or chicken there are **practically no carbs**.

Restaurants do seem to give us large meals, mostly padded out with the chips or potatoes, you may have to overcome lifelong habits here, of eating everything on your plate, however that thought process or conditioning does not serve you any more! Do not eat until you are so full you cannot move, stop when you have had enough, you will be surprised how good it feels to be in control. Just try it! Just remind yourself of your goals and of the work you have put in already, that you do not want to be wasted. Keep thinking protein and vegetables or protein and salad.

Alcohol however may be a problem, it is carbohydrate and should be limited. I personally have got used to topping up a small glass of dry white wine or red wine with water, this is about one or two grams of carbs and to me it still tastes like wine, alternatively drink water. Sweet wine or sparkling wine however is going to be around six to seven grams of carbs in each small glass of 125m. A half pint of beer or lager also has between five to seven grams of carbs so is probably not the best choice. You want to lose weight and get healthy and younger looking, that's worth a bit of sacrifice for a time isn't it?

Chapter 9: The Fat Switch at a glance Summary

Time to recap on the main points of The Fat Switch:

- Refined carbohydrates create high levels of Insulin

- High levels of Insulin cause excess carbohydrates to be parked as Fat especially around the waist and hips

- High levels of Insulin also make it difficult for the body to burn Fat

- If we lower our carbohydrate intake we lower our insulin levels.

- Then not only do we stop laying down so much fat but we activate our body to BURN BODY FAT as its first option for energy production!

- In the weight loss phase we limit our carbohydrate intake to around 50 grams per day.

- We follow the guides, keep a record of what we eat and check our progress after 7 days.

- We adjust our intake if necessary as we are all different and we keep going until we hit our desired weight.

- In the weight maintenance phase we can increase our carb intake to 100 grams per day, we still monitor our progress weekly.

- We use our new knowledge to improve our health and our diet has become normal to us.

- We enjoy our new weight, health and vitality!

Chapter 10: Easy portion guide

I promised that I would make this easy and I know its not always going to be possible to weigh your carbohydrates, this is an approximate and quick way to estimate the size of portions.

Make a fist and look down at it, this represents a portion for you personally (as your fist size is relative to your size). A mound on your plate, the size of your fist is one portion. This works for many foods like potatoes, chips, rice, pasta and many vegetables.

For dried foods and small grain foods prior to cooking again use your hand but this time open, a handful of uncooked rice (remember Basmati rice is best) or pasta or breakfast cereals should be measured in this simple way. Use your open hand also for nuts and dried fruit.

A portion of bread is one slice, wholegrain is best as it keeps you satisfied longer (see Chapter 15: Slow release food) and a bagel or large roll is two portions.

A portion of meat or fish is likely to be around 90 to 120 grams which is around the size of your open hand and not really any bigger. Remember you can have more of this!

A portion of butter or olive oil is 5 to 10 grams and in my view is preferable to fats and spreads even so called "healthy" ones (see Chapter 16: Healthy and essential oils).

A portion of cheese is around 40 grams, about the size of a match box approximately 2" x 3" x 1/2"(you can have more of this too).

My tip is stay relaxed, eat slowly, enjoy the food and the company if you are sharing a meal and do your best to stick to the portions.

Chapter 11: The Calorie Counting Myth

For over 50 years advice on losing weight has been based on cutting calories but it is pretty obvious that rates of obesity are rising. There has been plenty of research, in fact even as far back as 1971 The American Journal of Clinical Nutrition published details of a study carried out on young men of the same weight who dieted for 9 weeks. Their calorie intake was the same at1800 calories and they were split into 3 groups, each group was on either30 grams, 60 grams or 104 grams of carbohydrate per day. All of the groups lost weight but the low carb group lost the most and remember the calorie intake was the same. More surprisingly the **fat loss** in the low carb group was also much higher!

These studies demonstrate that low carbohydrate diets are better at helping you to lose weight and more importantly, to lose Fat. We also know that drastically cutting calories can cause the metabolism to slow, so it is important to eat regularly, particularly as your metabolism may take some time to get back to normal, even months!

As we have seen, different forms of calories react in the body in different ways, fast release (High GI) carbs cause a rush of Insulin, with results we do not want. What we want is to eat slow release(Low GI) carbs and limited intake which allows the body to process the resulting glucose effectively with no Fat being deposited.

Chapter 12: Barriers to Weight Loss

We know that being overweight is one of the biggest challenges facing the western world and that being overweight brings with it many serious medical conditions. So why can't we successfully lose weight and keep it off? Here are some of the common reasons why people give up:

1. It is too much effort to be dieting all the time

2. It's too complicated

3. I don't want to go without food and feel hungry

4. I don't want to spend hours in the gym

5. I can't afford fancy diet foods

6. Food makes me feel good

Don't worry if some of these might be you, that's now in the past, I am sharing with you something that should be common knowledge! The Fat Switch addresses these issues and increases your chances of success, here's how:

1. It is too much effort to be dieting all the time

You are not going to diet at all, just replace bad carbohydrates with nutritious alternatives, like protein and healthy fat.

2. It's too complicated

The Fat Switch is really simple you just try to Keep within your recommended guide line of carbohydrates each day.

3. I don't want to go without food and feel hungry

There is no reason to feel hungry, you will be switching to more tasty protein and healthy fat foods that fill, satisfy and provide excellent nutrition.

4. I don't want to spend hours in the gym

Me neither! In this book I will help you identify effective and easy exercise that you enjoy that suits you, like walking and Yoga.

5. I can't afford fancy diet foods

Ok, "diet foods" are usually low fat but high in carbohydrates in the form of sugar, which is the real problem. The Fat Switch gives you the true facts and moves you to better foods.

6. Food makes me feel good

Yes it does! But how good would you feel being healthier, looking good and being able to be more active? To support your state of mind The Fat Switch provides a chapter on relaxation techniques to help you de-stress and improve your sense of wellbeing.

I want it easy too! I can assure you that I follow this program myself and have made it, enjoyable, simple and straightforward, now I don't even have to think about it. What is more, as I follow this most of the time I can easily treat myself any time I want to, which often surprises people who are struggling with their weight. So enjoy your journey - I'm with you every step of the way!

Chapter 13: Your Diet and Your Health

When we use the words Weight Loss it tends to be misleading, many diets will create weight loss, unfortunately, when this weight loss is made up of muscle loss as well as fat loss and poor nutrition it can be bad for our health.

This book will inform and empower you to make easy, yet life changing nutrition and lifestyle decisions that decide the quality of life you are going to experience now and in the future! We need only to make some simple, well informed choices and our future changes dramatically!

Probably the biggest health related challenges facing us today are to avoid the many serious medical conditions brought on by poor diet and lifestyle. You do not need to accept many common yet serious medical conditions as inevitable with age and if we follow this simple program it is now possible to work towards a long, active and healthy life. Should we choose, using straight forward carbohydrate control, this legacy of good health and vitality can also be passed on to our friends and family.

This will be easy for you to adopt and will become the way you eat for life, ensuring a healthy weight and helping to avoid, manage or even eliminate the many medical conditions relating to being overweight.

There are many "fad" diets available but eliminating food groups entirely, fasting without change or simply reducing calories is not the way to lose weight, this book will guide you to balanced and improved nutrition, ensuring full vitality, health and wellbeing, based on sound medical evidence. Let's make this very clear, this is not just another diet book to try and then forget!

Armed with some simple knowledge you can easily maintain a healthy weight for life. I will fully advise you with clarity on both establish medical science and the latest nutritional and lifestyle research. It may not only involve you getting to a healthy weight, but can increase fitness, vitality and energy.

This book will change your life - maybe even save your life as losing weight can help to avoid or improve many life threatening medical conditions. You don't have to accept that things automatically go wrong as you get older and it is possible to live a long, active and healthy life, don't wait for things to go wrong then take medication, just do the right things now - you CAN do it!

Chapter 14: A New Level of Nutrition

I want to raise your level of nutrition to enable good health, in the weight maintenance phase you will be able to eat more carbs but those **carbs will be nutritious and slow release**. Whole grain carbs are exactly what they say! That is they contain the whole of the grain, especially the kernel which contains the nutrients we need. White, refined grains like white flour and white bread have had this removed so actually have no nutritional value to us. So you can already see that this simple change has many additional benefits!

Stop taking sweeteners now! Your body treats them just like sugar and they cause a rush of insulin or worse, read the chapter on sweeteners and slimming products for more information.

Fats have been blamed for increasing weight in the population however it is now widely accepted that our high intake of carbs is to blame. We will **increase our intake of healthy fats like olive oil and omega 3 fats**.

We lose muscle as we get older and if you have tried to lose weight before you have probably depleted muscle mass and bone density. To combat this we will increase protein and calcium intake at the same time by **eating larger portions of lean meat, oily fish, cheese and dairy**, this will replace some of the carbs we used to eat.

Fruit and vegetables are also essential to your health, they provide antioxidants, which help combat diseases such as cancer. They also provide fibre which keeps your digestive system healthy and helps to lower cholesterol, leafy green vegetables are excellent for reducing cholesterol levels.

Snacks may be necessary, but if you are hungry don't go for the refined carbs, nuts and seeds are a great choice and high in protein. They also provide many minerals and vitamins which help to protect us from illness and infection and they also help to keep up our energy levels. So snack on nuts and seeds rather than carbs.

I have provided more information on each of these food groups later in the book but for now here is the summary:

1. Throw the Fat Switch by dropping carb intake to around 50 grams per day and make those whole grain and slow release where possible.

2. Increase fruit and vegetables for essential minerals antioxidants and fibre.

3. Stop taking sweeteners they still create excess insulin.

4. Increase dairy intake for calcium to strengthen bones.

5. Increase good protein to build muscle (and bone).

6. Change to good fats to address any imbalance.

7. Limit treats to healthy choices like nuts and seeds for energy!

The above points are the main drive of the programme, in the next few chapters I will explain how to make more simple changes, not eating less but eating better! This will take your diet to the next really healthy level, watch out for life changes!

> **Motivation booster**
>
> You are dramatically improving
> your health whilst you lose
> weight on this plan!

Chapter 15: Slow release food

Different types of food release energy to the body at different rates, this is measured by something called the Glycemic Index (GI), all foods have a GI value. However we only need to know if foods are slow release or fast release.

This is particularly important with carbohydrates, bread, rice, pasta, cereals and potatoes. Brown or wholegrain varieties are generally slow release and therefore the best choice, in terms of rice, Basmati rice is also slow release and therefore a good choice. Additionally wholegrain is just what it says, it is the whole of the grain and contains the nutrition held in the kernel.

White varieties have been processed and the kernel and most useful fibre have been removed, reducing the nutritional value and turning them into fast release foods. Processed foods in general are more likely to have added sugars and fats and are likely to be fast release foods so where possible fresh foods are a better choice.

Most breakfast cereals, even the "healthy" ones are likely to be fast release foods and those little bits of dried "berries" just add to the sugar. The easiest way to check out the labels (if you want to) is to look under the 100grams column for "Carbohydrates of which sugars" and compare them like for like.

The best breakfast is porridge with a little dried fruit and flaked almonds or a couple of eggs on wholegrain toast. This is slow release food and should last you through to lunchtime without having to snack, but if you do snack try an apple or other fruit and a few nuts.

Chapter 16: Healthy and essential oils

I will give you the essential information you need to know about Omega 3, Omega 6 and Omega 9 oils and fats. Omega 9 is an unsaturated fatty acid which is found in olive oil and is predominant in the Mediterranean diet. The modern western diet is high in cheap animal and vegetable fats, these are usually Omega 6 fats, now the ideal balance between Omega 6 and Omega 3 is around 1 to 1 or 2 to 1. However because the primary sources of Omega 3 are oily fish or Hempseed and we don't eat either of these often enough most people will have a serious deficiency. This is made worse by the fact that Omega 6 is in almost everything processed (so we get lots of it) the actual imbalance therefore could be as high as 15 to 1.

Low levels of Omega 3 can cause circulation problems and inflammation of skin, glands and other organs. Omega 3 is essential for proper brain, bloodstream and nervous system function and can ease joint pain.

I would therefore recommend daily a supplement of good quality Omega 3 usually in the form of fish oil from a good source that is safe, balanced and mercury-free. If you are suffering from any of the above this could be a great improvement but check with your doctor first particularly if you are on medication.

Key Point
Supplement with Omega 3 fish oil for a wide range of benefits!

Chapter 17: Sweeteners and Slimming Products

Sweeteners

In a study carried out at Washington University, St Louis, on the effects of Splenda, a popular sucralose based sweetener, the sweetener was found to have an adverse effect on participant's blood sugar and insulin levels. They were given about as much as in one can of drink prior to being tested for glucose absorption.

Yanina Pepino PhD, the researcher summarised: "Everyone got the same amount of glucose, both times, but their bodies secreted much more insulin when they got sucralose first" .

"When study participants drank sucralose, their blood sugar peaked at a higher level than when they drank only water before consuming glucose. Insulin levels also rose about 20 % higher. So the artificial sweetener was related to an enhanced blood insulin and glucose response."

All sugar substitutes, including aspartame, sucralose, sorbitol and saccharin require your liver to do more work and can cause side effects. Although much research is disputed, there are many reports of side effects like headaches, fibromyalgia, anxiety, memory loss, arthritis, abdominal pain, nausea, depression, heart palpitations and irritable bowel syndrome, There is also initial concern that insulin is produced by the body in response to what it thinks is sugar, but it fails to find the sugar so issues even more insulin.

Our purpose is to reduce insulin and lose weight, you may be advised on balance to be cautious about sweeteners, in fact can anything claimed to be Zero that tastes sweet really be free?

Slimming Products

I have put Sweeteners and Slimming Products in the same chapter for two reasons:

1. Most slimming products are described as" Low Fat" or even "Zero Fat", don't be fooled, **weight loss is about the carbohydrates NOT the Fat.** Fifty years ago, when early research thought it was Fat that makes us Fat, the food industry went "Low Fat" , it effectively backed itself into a corner and it is still there.

    Fat and sugar are what make processed food taste good, so when they lowered the fat they often had to increase the sugar to keep any sort of taste. But adding sugar adds calories and Slimming Products have to be low calorie, (however we know it's not about the calories).So we come to point 2:

2. If the manufacturers haven't added extra sugar they will have added Sweeteners and on our healthy weight loss diet we don't want either sugar or sweeteners that cause over-production of insulin!

You do not need these slimming products, they will have an adverse effect on your insulin levels.

Always check for added sugar or sweeteners and remember fresh foods will not have added sugar!

> **Reminder**
>
> **Weight loss is about cutting**
> **carbohydrates not fat!**

Chapter 18: Processed versus fresh

Eating fresh food where possible will have a number of benefits. Fresh food is less likely to contain poor quality oils, fats or added sugar, salt and preservatives. Fresh food is also mostly going to be a slow release food which will benefit weight loss, frozen vegetables are ok but watch out for added sugar (carbohydrates). In addition processed foods often have added colours, preservatives and flavour enhancers, you can clean up your system by avoiding processed foods where possible and building up a repertoire of simple but tasty meals. The cost of fresh food is often raised as an objection but buying carefully when there are offers and choosing vegetables in season or on the market can help. You may eventually be able to change your view of food according to the nutrition it provides for you! Just four examples of cheap protein sources are baked beans, humous, red-skinned peanuts or tuna.

Chapter 19: Healthy lifestyle changes

I have made the case that just a small effort can deliver the desired results, so let's take a look at our lifestyle and see what other small changes might benefit us. Firstly how can we increase the amount of exercise we do? The government recommends 20 minutes a day of activity that increases our heart rate and makes us slightly breathless, this can be in shorter 10 minute bursts. Try to introduce these ideas but do consult your doctor if you are not used to exercise or have medical conditions:

Instead of ambling along when we walk try to increase the pace until we feel slightly breathless.

When using a car, park a little further from the shop, supermarket or other destination instead of as close as possible.

When using a bus get off one stop earlier and briskly walk to your destination or when catching a bus allow time to walk to the next stop and then catch the bus.

Always take the stairs instead of a lift and walk gently up escalators rather than standing still (these are big strides and give you a stretch).

Consider swimming or taking a course like yoga, pilates or dancing, one evening course is better than watching TV and may have sociable benefits too. Exercise also releases feel good chemicals in the body and reduces stress.

Chapter 20: Raise your mood and your game

Finally, losing weight, improving fitness and addressing nutritional gaps will make you feel better physically and mentally as your self-image improves and you have more energy to enjoy your new life.

Studies have shown that the psychological aspects relating to weight loss need to be addressed in addition to dietary changes if the programme is to be successful and if the weight loss is to be maintained. Most weight loss programmes don't do this and the results are often "yo-yo" dieting or even steadily increasing weight towards a very unhealthy weight.

So if you want to lose weight don't overlook your mind! Here are a few personal development techniques that we might introduce to feel even more relaxed and positive, to take our lives to a whole new level!

It has been said "You and your world are controlled by your thoughts. The wise person controls their thoughts". It is very common for people to be living a very stressful life, often the mind is full of unwanted negative thoughts, dwelling in the past or worrying about the future, the current moment is lost to us. We do not see the good things that present themselves every day, the trees, the sunshine the opportunity to smile, we can be lost in our thoughts and missing the current moment. We call this current moment "The Now" and I want to help your clear your mind and enjoy living in The Now.

If your mind is full of thoughts or worries try this simple exercise, close your eyes and imagine you are in a position inside your head, 3 or 4 inches behind your eyes. Imagine that you are looking at a screen and the thoughts are scrolling across the screen, gently clear the screen and enjoy the blank screen. Within seconds the thoughts are likely to return, when you notice that they are back gently clear the screen and enjoy the emptiness. Do this whenever you can and gradually the gaps between the thoughts will get longer and longer until you will find you have more peace. Worrying thoughts are just a habit, with gentle practice like this we can replace this habit giving us more time in the current moment.

The practice of Non Judgement can take a lifetime but taking every opportunity to practise can be very beneficial. Don't get drawn into negativity or criticism of others, if someone is being critical and is looking for you to reinforce their view be non-committal or simply move away. Seek out positive people and situations, make a point of noticing positive things like the sun, nature, animals etc and share this with others, be the positive person. You will find that you then encourage others around you to be positive too and you find that your thoughts have indeed created your world. Choose what you expose yourself to and limit your exposure to negativity like the news, your world is what you and your thoughts make it. Enjoy it, it's a great life!

Chapter 21: Conclusion

Well there it is, I hope you will agree that with very little effort in the right place and the right advice you really can lose weight, get in better shape and change your life. These changes should bring about weight loss of at least 1 to 2 pounds a week and as your body mass gets smaller simply reduce the portions in line with your weight. By the time you reach your desired weight this way, of eating and living, will have established itself as habit. You will finally be in control of your life, enjoying it without the pressure of worrying or dieting!

Quick and safe weight loss

One of the advantages of The 21st Century Fat Switch is the increased motivation of achieving quick results which really spurs people on to establish a great lifestyle change. Please feel free to contact me to discuss any problems or for support and advice.

For further support, discount nutrition, low carbohydrate meal replacement shakes, advice and articles please visit my websites and online shop at: **taowarrior.co.uk or alphapeople.co.uk**

Best Wishes for a Great Life

Mike Littlewood Dip GM, Dip SDT

"The 21st Century Fat Switch"

References

Effect of a Low-Carbohydrate Diet on Appetite, Blood Glucose Levels, and Insulin Resistance in Obese Patients with Type 2 Diabetes

Guenther Boden, MD; Karin Sargrad, MS, RD, CDE; Carol Homko, PhD, RN, CDE; Maria Mozzoli, BS; and T. Peter Stein, PhD

Systematic review and meta-analysis of clinical trials of the effects of low carbohydrate diets on cardiovascular risk factors. Obes Rev. 2012 Aug 21. doi: 10.1111/j.1467-789X.2012.01021.x.

Sucralose Affects Glycemic and Hormonal Responses to an Oral Glucose Load

M. Yanina Pepino, PHD, Courtney D. Tiemann, MPH, MS, RD,

Bruce W. Patterson, PHD, Burton M. Wice, PHD, Samuel Klein, MD

Effects of Diet-Induced Moderate Weight Reduction on Intrahepatic and Intramyocellular Triglycerides and Glucose Metabolism in Obese Subjects

Fumihiko Sato, Yoshifumi Tamura, Hirotaka Watada, Naoki Kumashiro, Yasuhiro Igarashi, Hiroshi Uchino, Tadayuki Maehara, Shinsuke Kyogoku, Satoshi Sunayama, Hiroyuki Sato, Takahisa Hirose, Yasushi Tanaka, and Ryuzo Kawamori